THE HIGH BLOOD PRESSURE CONTROL SECRET

A 6-Week Guide to Controlling Hypertension

Dr. BOB KENNETH

TABLE OF CONTENTS

INTRODUCTION

- The impact of diet on blood pressure.
- Introduction to the DASH (Dietary Approaches to Stop Hypertension) diet.
- The importance of staying hydrated for blood pressure control.

Chapter 4: Move Your Body, Calm Your Mind

Week 2 - Exercise and Stress Management:

- The role of physical activity in lowering blood pressure.
- Guided exercise routines for beginners.
- Stress reduction techniques and their impact on hypertension.

Chapter 5: Mastering Medication and Monitoring

Week 3 - Medication Management:

- Understanding prescribed medications.
- The importance of compliance and regular monitoring.

- Recognizing side effects and when to consult your healthcare provider.

Chapter 6: The Holistic Approach to Lasting Control

Weeks 4-6 - Integrating Holistic Strategies:

- The power of sleep in blood pressure control.
- Exploring alternative therapies such as yoga and meditation.
- Creating a long-term plan for maintaining healthy blood pressure levels.

Conclusion: Living a Heart-Healthy Life

Recap of the 6-week journey.

- Encouragement for a lifetime commitment to blood pressure management.
- Resources for ongoing support and education.

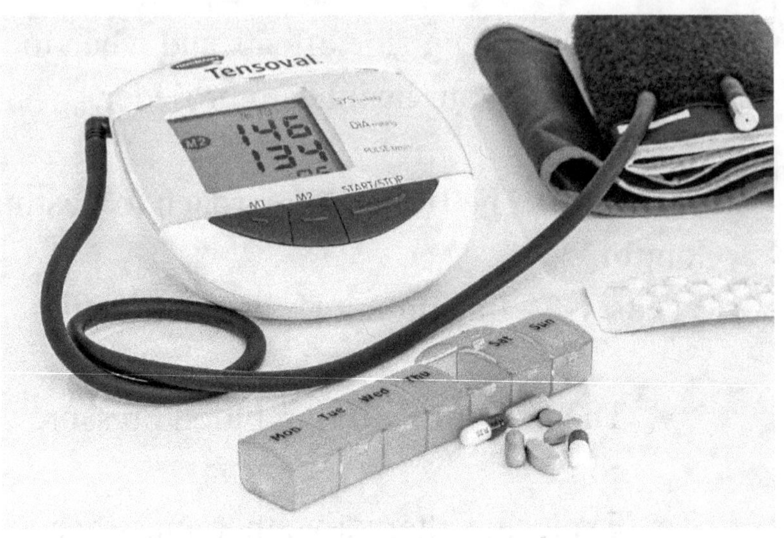

This book provides a comprehensive guide to understanding, managing, and controlling high blood pressure through a structured 6-week program. Each chapter focuses on a specific aspect of blood pressure control, offering practical tips, exercises, and advice to empower readers on their journey to a healthier, heart-conscious lifestyle.

INTRODUCTION TO HIGH BLOOD PRESSURE

In the quiet corridors of our bodies, a subtle danger often lurks, imperceptible to the naked eye but capable of wreaking havoc over time. High blood pressure, or hypertension, is a silent threat that affects millions worldwide, often going unnoticed until it manifests in severe health complications. This chapter aims to peel back the layers of this silent adversary, shedding light on what high blood pressure truly is and why it demands our attention.

Section 1: Defining Hypertension

- The Numbers Game:

Delve into the numerical indicators of blood pressure, breaking down the significance of systolic and diastolic readings.
Explore how blood pressure is measured and the accepted standards for defining hypertension.

- Understanding the Silent Nature:

Discuss the asymptomatic nature of high blood pressure and its ability to quietly damage organs over time.
Present real-life scenarios and stories to illustrate the hidden dangers of untreated hypertension.

Section 2: The Impact of Hypertension

- Beyond the Heart:

Examine how high blood pressure affects not only the heart but also various organs, including the kidneys, brain, and blood vessels. Illustrate the long-term consequences, such as stroke, heart attack, and kidney disease.

- Personalizing the Risk:

Identify the risk factors associated with hypertension, both modifiable and non-modifiable.
Encourage readers to assess their own risk and understand the importance of early intervention.

Section 3: The Call to Action

- Taking Control of Your Health:

Emphasize the significance of proactively managing blood pressure for overall well-being.
Motivate readers to embark on a journey towards blood pressure control.

- The Importance of Awareness:

Discuss the role of awareness campaigns, routine check-ups, and community engagement in tackling the silent epidemic.
Encourage readers to spread awareness within their communities and families.
By the end of this chapter, readers will have a profound understanding of the silent threat that is high blood pressure and will be motivated to take the necessary steps towards a healthier, more informed lifestyle.

CHAPTER 1
UNVEILING THE SILENT THREAT

- **Definition and understanding of hypertension**

Section 1: Defining Hypertension

- Definition and Understanding of Hypertension:

High blood pressure, medically known as hypertension, is a common cardiovascular condition characterized by elevated pressure within the arteries. To comprehend hypertension, it's crucial to break down the terminology and grasp the mechanics behind this silent threat.

- Deciphering Blood Pressure Readings:

Begin by explaining the two key components of blood pressure: systolic and diastolic.
Define systolic pressure as the force exerted on artery walls when the heart contracts, and diastolic pressure as the pressure between heartbeats when the heart is at rest.

- The Numbers Game:

Establish the normal range for blood pressure and distinguish between normal, prehypertension, and hypertension readings.
Illustrate how blood pressure is measured using a sphygmomanometer, emphasizing the importance of accurate readings.

- Understanding the Silent Nature:

Unveil the insidious nature of hypertension by explaining its asymptomatic characteristics.

Clarify that, unlike overt symptoms, hypertension often operates in the background, silently damaging arteries and vital organs.

Section 2: The Impact of Hypertension

- Beyond the Numbers:

Expand the definition by exploring the broader impact of hypertension on overall health.
Discuss how elevated blood pressure affects the delicate balance of the cardiovascular system, leading to complications such as atherosclerosis and organ damage.

- Risk Factors and Causes:

Identify common risk factors for hypertension, including age, genetics, lifestyle choices, and underlying health conditions.
Emphasize the multifaceted nature of hypertension, where a combination of genetic predisposition and environmental factors can contribute to its development.

- The Vicious Cycle:

Illustrate the feedback loop of hypertension, where sustained high blood pressure further damages arteries, leading to a continuous cycle of cardiovascular stress.

Emphasize the urgency of breaking this cycle through intervention and lifestyle changes. Understanding hypertension involves not just recognizing the numerical values but also appreciating its systemic effects on the body. As readers delve into this definition, they lay the foundation for comprehending the intricacies of blood pressure and its impact on overall health.

- The silent dangers of untreated high blood pressure and the importance of taking control for a healthier life.

High blood pressure, or hypertension, is not merely a numerical anomaly on a medical chart; it's a silent saboteur, capable of inflicting severe damage when left unchecked. In this section, we unravel the quiet dangers that untreated high blood pressure poses and emphasize the pivotal role of taking control for a healthier life.

- Understanding the Silent Nature:

The Silent Dangers of Untreated High Blood Pressure:

Examine how hypertension, if left unmanaged, silently targets vital organs like the heart, kidneys, brain, and blood vessels.
Detail the cascading effects of sustained high pressure, contributing to the development of serious conditions such as heart disease, stroke, and kidney failure.

- Subtle Symptoms, Serious Consequences:

Shed light on the absence of overt symptoms in the early stages, allowing hypertension to operate stealthily.
Illustrate through real-life examples how the lack of immediate symptoms may lead individuals to underestimate the urgency of

managing their blood pressure.

- **The Impact of Hypertension**

The Importance of Taking Control for a Healthier Life:

Preventing the Domino Effect:

Emphasize the domino effect of untreated hypertension, where damage to one organ sets off a chain reaction affecting the entire cardiovascular system.
Highlight the role of proactive blood pressure management in preventing this cascade of health issues.

- Quality of Life Matters:

Discuss how untreated hypertension can significantly reduce one's quality of life, impacting daily activities and overall well-being.
Encourage readers to envision a life unburdened by the silent threats of

hypertension, motivating them to take charge of their health.
Connection Between Silent Dangers and Taking Control:

- Empowering Change:

Stress the empowering aspect of taking control – a conscious decision to break free from the silent dangers of untreated hypertension. Share success stories of individuals who, through lifestyle changes and medical intervention, reclaimed control of their health and reversed the damaging effects of high blood pressure.

- The Wellness Journey:

Conclude by reinforcing the idea that taking control of hypertension is not just a medical obligation but a journey towards a healthier, more fulfilling life.
Set the stage for the chapters ahead, which will guide readers through a transformative 6-week

program aimed at lowering blood pressure and securing a healthier future.

By understanding the silent dangers of untreated high blood pressure and recognizing the importance of taking control, readers are prepared to embark on a journey of self-discovery and proactive health management.

CHAPTER 2

KNOW YOUR NUMBERS AND INTERPRET BLOOD PRESSURE READINGS

describing blood pressure's systolic and diastolic values.

understanding the meaning of the numbers on a blood pressure measurement.

Recognizing risk variables and appreciating individual risk

- Comprehending Blood Pressure Measurements:

Anyone trying to control hypertension must be able to navigate the maze of blood pressure measurements. We will explore the nuances of blood pressure in this chapter, helping readers understand the statistics and make sense of their readings. The first step to taking charge is to comprehend the subtle differences between systolic and diastolic blood pressure.

1. Systolic and diastolic blood pressure explanation:

Systolic Blood Pressure:

Systolic pressure is the force that the heart applies to the artery walls during a heartbeat, pumping blood into the bloodstream. Demonstrate how systolic pressure affects cardiovascular health overall and is important for evaluating the heart's effectiveness.

Diastolic Blood Pressure:

Diastolic pressure is defined as the pressure within the arteries during the period between heartbeats.

Stress that diastolic pressure is a vital sign of the general health of the vascular system since it represents the resistance in the arteries.

2. How to Interpret Readings of Blood Pressure:

- Interpreting the Numbers:

Normal versus High:

Determine the normal blood pressure standard range.

Explain high blood pressure and its effects, emphasizing the value of prompt treatment.

- High blood pressure and prehypertension:

Talk about the cutoff points that distinguish between pre-hypertensive and hypertensive blood pressure phases.

Give concise explanations of the implications of each step for the health and welfare of the individual.

- Comprehending Variability

Describe how the blood pressure naturally varies during the day.
Assist readers in understanding what they read for themselves, taking the time of day and previous activities into account.

3. Determining Risk Elements and Comprehending Individual Risk:

- Above and Beyond the Stats:

Changeable Risk Elements

Examine the lifestyle variables that affect blood pressure, such as nutrition, exercise, and stress reduction.
Give doable advice on how to improve everyday living and lower changeable risk factors.

- Non-Adaptable Risk Elements:

Talk about age, family history, and genetic predisposition as non-modifiable risk factors. Assist readers in comprehending how proactive health measures may successfully handle these circumstances, even when they are beyond their control.

- Evaluating Individual Risk:

Provide instruments for evaluating individual risk that take into account both changeable and unchangeable elements.
Urge readers to consult candidly with medical professionals to develop individualized blood pressure control strategies.
There is more to understanding blood pressure readings than just the numbers. It gives people the ability to see trends, evaluate their risk factors, and decide with knowledge for a healthy future. Equipped with this understanding, readers are ready for the next chapters, which will walk them through doable actions to bring their blood pressure down.

CHAPTER 3
THE INFLUENCE OF LIFESTYLE ADJUSTMENTS

Week 1: Intentional Consumption and Drinking:

Dietary influences on blood pressure.
An overview of the DASH diet, or Dietary Approaches to Stop Hypertension.
The value of maintaining hydration in managing blood pressure.

- Hydration and Mindful Eating

Using lifestyle modifications as a transforming tool is essential when starting the path to treat high blood pressure. We go into the topics of mindful eating and hydration in Week 1 and examine the significant effects these decisions may have on blood pressure.

1. Dietary Influence on Blood Pressure:

- Recognizing the Link Between Culinary and The Dilemma of Sodium:

Explain the connection between high blood pressure and salt consumption.
Assist readers in locating hidden sodium sources in their food and in making decisions that will lower their salt intake.
The Paradox of Potassium:

Describe how potassium helps to maintain healthy blood pressure and balance salt.

Present foods high in potassium and stress how they should be a part of a diet that promotes heart health.

Wonderful Munchies:

Highlight certain items, such as leafy greens, berries, and nuts, that are known to decrease blood pressure.
Provide useful advice on how to include these items in regular meals.

2. Overview of the DASH Nutrition Plan:

- A Nutritional Strategy to Lower Blood Pressure:

Basics of the DASH Diet:

Give a brief explanation of the DASH diet's scientific basis for lowering blood pressure.
Dissect the essential elements, putting special attention on whole grains, dairy, fruits, and vegetables, as well as lean proteins.

Useful DASH:

Provide exemplary menus and dishes that adhere to the DASH diet guidelines.
Dispel typical misunderstandings and difficulties while offering answers that are simple to implement.

Prolonged Devotion:

Stress the DASH diet's durability as a long-term lifestyle option.
Urge readers to consider dietary modifications as a component of a comprehensive strategy for managing blood pressure.

3. The Need for Maintaining Hydration to Regulate Blood Pressure:

- Satisfying Your Thirst for Improved Health

Blood pressure and water:

Describe how consuming enough water helps to maintain normal blood pressure levels.

Dispel the rumors about staying hydrated and highlight the health advantages of water as the best calorie-free beverage.

Drinking Routines:

Give helpful advice on how to maintain hydration throughout the day, such as establishing hydration regimens and including meals high in water.
Describe difficulties and provide solutions for typical obstacles to sustaining enough hydration.

Past the Water

Investigate substitute, heart-healthy drinks that provide general hydration without jeopardizing blood pressure regulation.
Reciterate the connection between better cardiovascular health and careful hydration.
In addition to learning the immediate effects of mindful eating and staying hydrated on blood pressure, readers who begin Week 1 of lifestyle adjustments will also establish the groundwork

for long-term dietary practices that support a heart-healthy lifestyle.

CHAPTER 4
EXERCISE YOUR BODY, RELAX YOUR THOUGHTS

Week 2: Physical Activity and Stress Reduction

- The impact of exercise on blood pressure reduction.
- workout regimens with guidance for novices.
- The effects of stress management strategies on hypertension.

In **Week 2**, we explore the dynamic pair of exercise and stress reduction, revealing their mutual benefits for blood pressure regulation. The transforming potential of movement for the body and mind will become clear to readers as we examine the impact of exercise and stress-reduction practices.

1. The Function of Exercise in Blood Pressure Reduction:

- Realizing Movement's Potential:

Heart Rate and Arterial Condition:

Describe how engaging in regular exercise improves blood flow artery health and flexibility.
Provide evidence of the direct relationship between exercise and lowered blood pressure.

Resistance vs. Aerobic Training:

Make a distinction between resistance and aerobic training, emphasizing each type's special benefits for heart health.
Give instructions on how to combine the two kinds of workouts into a comprehensive fitness regimen.

Duration, Intensity, and Frequency:

Talk about the ideal blood pressure control guidelines for exercise frequency, duration, and intensity.

Adapt the instructions to the different levels of fitness so that readers may discover a regimen that works for them.

2. Beginner-Friendly Guided Exercise Programs:

- From Passive to Intense:

Laying the Groundwork:

Introduce beginner-friendly workouts that are easy to do and effective.
Give detailed directions for fundamental exercises to progressively build up your strength and stamina.

Both indoors and outside:

Provide a variety of exercises that can be done outside or at home.
Include alternatives that don't require any equipment so that readers with a variety of fitness resources may access them.
Monitoring Progress:

Stress the value of monitoring your progress to maintain motivation.
Describe methods and instruments for tracking alterations in fitness levels throughout time.

3. Stress Reduction Methods and How They Affect Blood Pressure:

- Quieting the Inner Storm:

Recognizing the Relationship Between Stress and Blood Pressure:

Examine the physiological connection between high blood pressure and stress.
Inform readers about the long-term effects of prolonged stress on high blood pressure.

Mind-Body Methodologies:

Describe deep breathing techniques, meditation, and mindfulness as useful skills for reducing stress.

Give detailed directions on how to apply these methods in your day-to-day activities.

Comprehensive Methods:

Highlight holistic methods of reducing stress, such as progressive muscular relaxation and yoga.
Showcase how these techniques improve general mental and physical health in addition to reducing stress.
Readers will see firsthand the significant effects of exercise and stress reduction on blood pressure as they immerse themselves in Week 2. This chapter establishes the foundation for a comprehensive strategy to control hypertension via physical and mental well-being, including guided exercises and soothing techniques.

CHAPTER 5
MASTERING MEDICATION AND MONITORING

Week 3 - Medication Management

Recognizing the effects of prescription drugs. the significance of frequent monitoring and compliance.
Identifying adverse effects and knowing when to contact your doctor

Week 3 of our blood pressure control journey presents us with the topic of medication's involvement in managing hypertension. This chapter provides readers with the information they need to comprehend prescription drugs, emphasizes the value of following instructions, and describes the relevance of routine monitoring for a thorough approach to blood pressure control.

1. Recognizing Prescription Drugs:

- Cracking the Code of Medication:

Typical Classifications of Blood Pressure Drugs:

Give a summary of the drugs that are frequently prescribed to treat hypertension, such as beta-blockers, diuretics, ACE inhibitors, and calcium channel blockers. Describe the mechanism of action of each blood pressure-lowering drug.

Tailored Care Programs:

Stress how individualized hypertension therapy is.
To understand the reasoning behind the selected drugs and any potential revisions, readers are encouraged to have open contact with their healthcare practitioners.

2. The Significance of Consistency and Frequent Inspection:

- Creating a Successful Consistency:

Following prescription regimens:

Emphasize how important adherence is to obtaining the best possible blood pressure management.
Talk about typical obstacles to compliance and provide workable solutions.

The Function of Consistent Monitoring

Stress how important it is to regularly check your blood pressure at home and when seeing the doctor.
Advise on how to choose and use a home blood pressure monitor.
Reactions Close the Loop with Medical Providers:

Promote frequent check-ins with medical professionals to discuss possible modifications and the effectiveness of prescribed medications.
Emphasize that managing hypertension is a collaborative process that involves patients and

healthcare providers working together to get the greatest results.

3. Identifying Adverse Reactions and Knowing When to Contact Your Medical Professional:

- Getting Around the Drug Landscape:

Typical Adverse Reactions:

Describe any possible adverse effects that may arise from using blood pressure medication. Give readers the ability to distinguish between responses that are expected and those that need to be addressed right away.
Emergency Conditions and Warning Signs:

Teach readers how to spot serious side effects or blood pressure medication crises.
Give precise instructions on when to seek emergency medical treatment.
Maintain Open Channels of Communication:

Emphasize how crucial it is to keep lines of communication open with medical professionals about any worries or changes in your health.

Promote taking a proactive stance when it comes to managing side effects and making sure that the recommended drugs are in line with your overall health objectives.

Readers will acquire the skills and self-assurance necessary to successfully negotiate the complicated world of hypertension drugs as they participate in **Week 3.** By encouraging proactive medication management and monitoring, people advance in their quest to become experts at controlling their blood pressure

CHAPTER 6
A COMPREHENSIVE STRATEGY FOR DURABLE CONTROL

As we reach the last phase of our blood pressure management journey, we shift to a comprehensive strategy that combines many components into a long-term, sustainable plan. The reader will examine the relationship between sleep, complementary treatments, and long-term planning for long-term blood pressure control in this chapter, which focuses on Weeks 4 through 6.

1. Sleep's Influence on Blood Pressure Regulation:

- Unlocking the Benefits of Restorative

Circadian Rhythms and Sleep:

Analyze the connection between blood pressure control, circadian cycles, and sleep patterns.

Stress how crucial getting a good night's sleep is to maintaining cardiovascular health in general.

- Developing Restful Sleep Routines:

Give helpful advice on how to create sleep-promoting behaviors and enhance sleep hygiene.
Talk about how maintaining regular sleep patterns and nighttime rituals helps to maintain ideal blood pressure.

2. Examining Complementary Medicines:

- Various Paths to Wellbeing:

For Mind-Body Harmony, Yoga:

Describe yoga as a comprehensive discipline that incorporates breathing exercises, physical postures, and meditation.
Examine particular yoga positions and practices that have been shown to lower blood pressure.

Mindfulness & Meditation:

Explore the advantages of mindfulness and meditation for lowering blood pressure and reducing stress.
Give readers some guided meditation activities to add to their everyday routines.

3. Formulating a Long-Term Strategy to Keep Blood Pressure at Healthy Levels:

- The seeds of enduring change

The Use of Lifestyle as Medicine:

Reiterate the notion that maintaining blood pressure management requires making lifestyle decisions.
Urge readers to see their improved behaviors as a permanent commitment to health rather than as a short-term solution.

- Regular Evaluations of Health:

Emphasize the value of routine health examinations for both monitoring blood pressure and general well-being.
Promote early intervention and proactive health management.

- Systems of Community and Support:

Emphasize how important support networks and community involvement are to sustaining motivation.
Urge readers to talk to friends, relatives, or support groups about their struggles, triumphs, and experiences.

CONCLUSION

Maintaining Heart Health

- Honoring the Journey:

Considering the Advancement:

Encourage readers to consider the advancements they have achieved throughout the last six weeks.
Honor accomplishments, no matter how minor, and recognize the effort put out to maintain long-term blood pressure management.
Accepting a Future with Heart Health:

List the essential components of a comprehensive strategy for controlling blood pressure.
Encourage readers to embrace a heart-healthy future by emphasizing that they have the power to take long-term control.
By the time this trip ends, readers will have developed a holistic mentality that takes into

account all the interrelated aspects of their well-being in addition to learning how to regulate their blood pressure. They can live a heart-healthy life for many years to come as they go forward.

Weeks 4–6: Including Holistic Approaches

The ability of sleep to regulate blood pressure. investigating complementary therapies like yoga and meditation.
creating a long-term strategy to keep blood pressure readings in a reasonable range.

Weeks 4 through **6** of our blood pressure control program are the last phase, and as such, we will be concentrating on holistic strategies—tying together disparate components for a complete approach to long-term well-being. Readers will investigate the life-changing effects of restorative sleep, and holistic therapies like yoga and meditation, and create a customized, long-term plan to keep blood pressure levels in check throughout this time.

1. Sleep's Influence on Blood Pressure
Regulation:

- Setting Sleep First for Vitality:

Comprehending Sleep Cycles:

Examine the phases of sleep and how they aid
in the promotion of both mental and physical
healing.
Draw attention to the relationship between
blood pressure management and sleep cycles.

- Blood pressure and the length of sleep:

Talk about the ideal amount of time to sleep to
keep your blood pressure levels in check.
Examine the effects on cardiovascular health of
both too little and too much sleep.
Establishing a Setting That Promotes Sleep:

Give helpful advice on how to improve the
sleeping environment, taking into account

things like noise reduction, darkened rooms, and cozy bedding.
Encourage your body to signal for rest by establishing a pre-sleep routine.

2. Examining Complementary Medicines:

- Various Paths to Wellbeing:

For Mind-Body Harmony, Yoga:

Provide some more yoga poses that go well with the ones you learned in Week 2.
Stress the many health advantages of yoga, such as increased flexibility, lowered stress levels, and better general well-being.
Mindfulness and Meditation Techniques:

Extend the previously taught meditation skills by offering more complex methods for increased concentration and relaxation.
Give your thoughts on how to incorporate mindfulness into your everyday life to manage stress over time.

3. Formulating a Long-Term Strategy to Keep Blood Pressure at Healthy Levels:

- The seeds of enduring change

The Foundation of Lifestyle:

Reiterate the notion that maintaining blood pressure management is mostly dependent on lifestyle decisions.
Urge readers to consider their journey thus far and determine which lifestyle modifications have yielded the greatest results.

- Regular Evaluations of Health:

Emphasize the value of routine medical exams for ongoing blood pressure monitoring.
Advise on how to keep lines of communication open with medical professionals so that you may discuss changes in lifestyle and treat any new issues that may arise.

- Individualized Wellness Plan:

Help readers create a customized long-term
plan that incorporates effective lifestyle
modifications.
Promote the establishment of precise
objectives, reasonable deadlines, and plans for
resolving any obstacles.

Concluding the Matter: Leading a Heart-Well
Life

Accepting the Trip Ahead:

Recognizing Development:

Celebrate the victories and benchmarks attained
over the six-week course of the program.
Reiterate the notion that even modest positive
adjustments lead to long-term well-being.
Investing in the Future of Heart Health:

Write a summary of the holistic techniques you
acquired in the course.
Encourage readers to keep up their dedication
to a heart-healthy lifestyle by reassuring them

that they have the means to maintain blood pressure management.

By the time readers finish this extensive program, they will have adopted a holistic lifestyle that supports general health and wellbeing in addition to having the information necessary to properly manage their blood pressure. The trip comes to an end, but the inspiration to lead a heart-healthy life never goes away.

Summary of the six-week excursion. encouragement to maintain blood pressure control throughout one's life.

Reviewing the major turning points and lessons learned over the life-changing six-week journey to blood pressure control is crucial. Every week provided fresh insights, useful tactics, and a greater comprehension of how all-encompassing methods might result in long-lasting control. Let's review the key components of this journey:

Week 1: Exposing the Quiet Danger

examined the hidden risks associated with untreated high blood pressure.
emphasized how crucial it is to take charge to live a better life.
Described, along with its effects on key organs and the link between knowledge and preventive care.

Week 2: Recognize Your Pixels

divided blood pressure measurements into diastolic and systolic halves.
interpreted blood pressure readings and determined potential risk variables.
urged readers to become aware of their own risk of hypertension.

Week 3: The Influence of Modified Lifestyles

examined how nutrition affects blood pressure and presented the DASH diet.
emphasized how crucial staying hydrated is to controlling blood pressure.

started the process of adopting a more conscious diet and lifestyle.

Week 4: Get Moving, Relax Your Mind

highlighted how exercise may help reduce blood pressure.
provide beginner-friendly fitness regimens with guidance.
introduced mindfulness and exercise as ways to relieve stress.

Week 5: Getting the Hang of Medication and Tracking

clarified the prescription drug knowledge for hypertension.
emphasized the significance of frequent monitoring and compliance.
spoke about identifying adverse effects and when to contact medical professionals.

Weeks 4–6: Including Holistic Approaches

investigated how sleep affects blood pressure regulation.
explored complementary therapy such as yoga and meditation.
promoted the development of a long-term strategy for preserving normal blood pressure levels.
Motivating Individuals to Make a Lifelong Dedicated to Blood Pressure Control

Recall that managing your blood pressure is a lifelong commitment as you wrap up your six-week trip. Your commitment, consciousness, and proactive decisions have made the way for a more vibrant, healthy future. Here are some inspiring words:

- Honor accomplishments:

No matter how tiny the improvements you've made, be proud of them.
Honor your dedication to acquiring and applying health-promoting techniques.
Welcome to Consistency

Understand that maintaining a consistent lifestyle calls for a lifetime commitment. Consider every day as a chance to reaffirm good practices that help regulate blood pressure.

- Remain Up to Date:

Maintain your knowledge of hypertension, recent findings, and changing approaches to better blood pressure control.
You can make more educated decisions regarding your health when you are well-informed.

- Activate the Support Systems:

Tell your story to loved ones, support networks, and friends.
Be in the company of people who support and inspire you in your efforts to lead a heart-healthy lifestyle.

- Frequent Medical Examinations:

Continue to monitor your blood pressure and
get frequent health check-ups.
Communicate openly with your healthcare
professionals, revealing any concerns you may
have and updating them on your progress.

- Flexibility and Adaptability:

Recognize that situations may change and that
life is dynamic.
Be flexible and modify your tactics as
necessary to account for various stages of life.

- Consider Your Progress:

Review your trip regularly, noting your
accomplishments as well as your room for
growth.
Utilize this insight to improve and hone your
blood pressure control strategy over time.
Keep in mind that this journey is about
investing in your complete well-being rather
than merely controlling your blood pressure.
Your dedication now creates the groundwork
for a happier, healthier tomorrow. With the

information and resources at your disposal, you may confidently take on the future and live a heart-healthy life for many years to come.

www.ingramcontent.com/pod-product-compliance
Lightning Source LLC
Chambersburg PA
CBHW070213260726
48658CB00006BA/2068